Why **Magnesium** Is **the Key to Long-Term Health**

Other books by this author

- **Microscopic Colitis**
- **Understanding Microscopic Colitis**
- **Vitamin D and Autoimmune Disease**
- **8 Ways to Prevent Pancreatic Cancer**

Why Magnesium Is the Key to Long-Term Health

by Wayne Persky

Persky Farms

United States

First published and distributed in the United States of America by:
Persky Farms, 19242 Darrs Creek Rd, Bartlett, TX 76511-4460. Tel.: (1)254-718-1125; Fax: (1)254-527-3682. www.perskyfarms.com

Copyright: This book is protected under the US Copyright Act of 1976, as amended, and all other applicable international, federal, state, and local laws. All rights reserved. No part of this book may be reproduced by any mechanical, photographic, or electronic process, or in the form of an audio recording, nor may it be transmitted or otherwise copied for public or private use, other than the "fair use" purposes allowed by copyright law, without prior written permission of the publisher.

Disclaimer and Legal Notice: The information contained in this book is intended solely for general educational purposes, and is not intended, nor implied, to be a substitute for professional medical advice relative to any specific medical condition or question. The advice of a physician or other health care provider should always be sought for any questions regarding any medical condition. Specific diagnoses and therapies can only be provided by the reader's physician. Any use of the information in this book is at the reader's discretion. The author and the publisher specifically disclaim any and all liability arising directly or indirectly from the use or application of any information contained in this book.

Please note that much of the information in this book is based on personal experience and anecdotal evidence. Although the author and publisher have made every reasonable attempt to achieve complete accuracy of the content, they assume no responsibility for errors or omissions. If you should choose to use any of this information, use it according to your best judgment, and at your own risk. Because your particular situation will not exactly match the examples upon which this information is based, you should adjust your use of the information and recommendations to fit your own personal situation.

This book does not recommend or endorse any specific tests, products, procedures, opinions, or other information that may be mentioned anywhere in the book. This information is provided for educational purposes, and reliance on any tests, products, procedures, or opinions mentioned in the book is solely at the reader's own risk.

Any trademarks, service marks, product names, or named features are assumed to be the property of their respective owners, and are used only for reference. There is no implied endorsement when these terms are used in this book.

Copyright © Wayne Persky, 2018. All rights reserved worldwide.

ISBN 978-1-7328220-0-9

"There are only two ways to live your life. One is as though nothing is a miracle. The other is as though everything is a miracle." - Albert Einstein

Contents

Introduction...IX

Chapter 1...1
    What is magnesium and why is it important?

Chapter 2...9
    Why Have so Many of Us Become Magnesium Deficient?

Chapter 3...21
    How Accurate Are the Magnesium Tests Usually Used by Doctors?

Chapter 4...31
    What Types of Magnesium Are Available for Use as a Supplement?

Chapter 5...39
    What Else Should We Know About Magnesium?

About the Author..55

References...59

Introduction

To say that magnesium is important for health is a huge understatement. Besides being a vital electrolyte that is responsible for regulating the heart, lungs, and most other organs that are critical for life, magnesium is required for co-activating over 300 chemical processes in the body that are necessary for normal daily life. If we were to try to select one single element that is most important for good health, arguably, it would be magnesium.

In an article describing the importance of magnesium, Dr. Mark Sircus pointed out that Dr. Norman Shealy, a well-known neurosurgeon and pioneer in the development of pain medicine, once noted that "Every known illness is associated with a magnesium deficiency" (Sircus, 2009, December 8).[1] Furthermore, Dr. Shealy added that "magnesium is the most critical mineral required for electrical stability of every cell in the body. A magnesium deficiency may be responsible for more diseases than any other nutrient."

As Dr. Mark Sircus points out, a magnesium deficiency can cause any of the following symptoms

- abnormal heart rhythms
- agoraphobia
- angina

Why Magnesium Is the Key to Long-Term Health

- an inability to control the bladder
- anxiety
- a peculiar sensation that one needs to take a deep breath but can't
- apprehensiveness
- back aches
- blurry vision that changes from day to day
- chest tightness
- constipation
- coronary spasms
- difficulty swallowing or a lump in the throat
- dry, itchy skin
- extreme hunger
- extreme thirst
- fatigue
- foot pain
- frequent or recurring skin, gum, bladder or vaginal yeast infections
- frequent urination
- hearing loss
- heart arrhythmias
- high blood pressure
- hyperactivity and restlessness with constant movement
- hyper-excitability
- insomnia
- irritability
- jaw joint dysfunction (TMJ)
- leg cramps
- loss of appetite
- menstrual cramps

Introduction

- mitral valve prolapse
- muscle soreness
- muscle tension
- muscle twitches or spasms
- nausea
- neck pain
- noise sensitivity
- numbness
- nystagmus (rapid eye movements)
- osteoporosis
- palpitations
- panic attacks
- personality changes
- premenstrual irritability
- seizures
- sores or bruises that heal slowly
- tension headaches
- tingling
- twitches
- unexplained weight loss
- unusual tiredness or drowsiness
- urinary spasms
- vomiting
- weakness

It's interesting to note that the symptoms of severe magnesium deficiency are also common symptoms of diabetes or what's known as prediabetes. As we shall see later, this isn't merely a coincidence.

Why Magnesium Is the Key to Long-Term Health

Magnesium is important to all forms of life. For example, chlorophyll, the substance that gives plants their green color, contains magnesium.

And taking an appropriate magnesium supplement can eliminate any of the symptoms on that list (if they are caused by a magnesium deficiency, rather than something else).

The primary purpose of this book, then, is to define when it is appropriate to take a magnesium supplement, what type of supplement to take, and how much to take.

Chapter 1

What is Magnesium and Why Is It so Important?

As mentioned in the introduction, magnesium is vital not only for our long-term health, but also for our daily quality of life.

Excluding any chaotic events, our long-term health is primarily determined by three factors — our diet, the atmosphere around us, and the level of stress that pervades our lives. Of these three, normally our diet has the most pronounced effect by far on our health, but the air and any pollutants it contains may also have an important effect as we breathe it and it enter our bodies by absorption through our skin. And of course stress is the wild card that can have an effect that ranges from minor to dominant.

Magnesium may seem like an insignificant part of our diet since the actual amount needed is such a very small percentage of our diet. But its importance to our health is all out of proportion

Why Magnesium Is the Key to Long-Term Health

when compared with any other item in our diet except water and air (if you choose to consider air and water a part of our diet).

Magnesium is a gray-colored solid. It's a chemical element that appears in the periodic table with the atomic number 12. Magnesium is designated as Mg. It's an electrolyte, meaning that it produces an electrically conducting solution when dissolved in certain solvents, including blood serum. This allows it to facilitate many chemical reactions in the body.

One of the most important chemical processes is the activation of certain vitamins, so that the body can use them. Vitamin D, for example, is used by the immune system to fight infection, cancer, and disease in general. Without activated vitamin D, the ability of the immune system to defend the body and to promote healing is severely compromised.

As noted in the introduction, magnesium is used as a cofactor for converting the inactive form of vitamin D into the active form. Published data tells us that if magnesium supplies are inadequate, the human body will be unable to utilize vitamin D, because it will be unable to convert it from 25-hydroxyvitamin D [25(OH)D] into the active form of 1,25-dihydroxyvitamin D [1,25-(OH)2D] so that it can be used to fight inflammation and do all the other wonderful things attributed to vitamin D (Reddy & Sivakumar, 1974, Rude et al., 1985).[2,3] This is old research, but it provides valuable basic information and this particular attribute is vitally important for healing and long-term health.

What is Magnesium and Why Is It so Important?

Unfortunately, medical professionals often seem to completely ignore it today.

This probably defines why some patients (who have various diseases) are unable to properly heal. And it explains why some people are able to heal much faster than others. Healing is severely compromised if the patient has a magnesium deficiency. If the deficiency is bad enough, complete recovery may be impossible despite meticulous attention to other treatment details. This clearly illuminates why an adequate magnesium level is so important when one is attempting to recover from any disease or some other challenge to our immune system.

Magnesium is not just another nutrient.
As we have already discussed in this chapter, magnesium is an electrolyte that's absolutely essential for the completion of many essential processes required continually by many of the systems that allow the human body to function normally. Magnesium helps to regulate our heart rate, our breathing, our blood pressure, and our body temperature, among other things, so it's no wonder that it's so important for our long-term health.

Here are some additional examples of why it's so important for all of us to maintain adequate levels of magnesium.

Magnesium deficiency is associated with the development of insulin resistance and type 2 diabetes.

Takaya, Higashino, and Kobayashi (2004) showed that both hypertension and type 2 diabetes involve low magnesium levels in the cells of the body.[4]   In that research article, Takaya, Higashino, and Kobayashi (2004) concluded that because magnesium is necessary in order for the body to be able to use glucose properly, and magnesium is also used for insulin signaling, a deficiency of magnesium in the cells may alter the availability of glucose and thereby contribute to the development of insulin resistance.

In other words, magnesium and insulin are co-dependent.

Not only is magnesium deficiency associated with hypertension, but if the availability or either one (magnesium or insulin) is less than adequate, there is a much grater risk of developing diabetes or a condition known as pre-diabetes. Insulin is responsible for transporting nutrients out of the bloodstream to locations in the cells of the body where they can either be used immediately or stored for future use. A magnesium deficiency can not only cause insulin resistance (in the cells of the body), but it can cause reduced insulin production by the pancreas. And this in turn has a reciprocal effect — when the availability and effectiveness of insulin is compromised, extra magnesium in the blood cannot be properly stored, so most of it may be wasted, instead (Sircus, 2009).[5]

What is Magnesium and Why Is It so Important?

Obviously, this can become a self-perpetuating process. Once it starts, it can rather quickly lead to a condition that predisposes to diabetes. And once someone is caught in this spiral, it becomes more and more difficult for that individual to absorb magnesium, which makes the situation progressively worse.

Even stronger evidence of the association between magnesium deficiency and diabetes has been found by other researchers. Research published by Hruby et al. (2014) showed that people who have higher magnesium intake levels have a significantly lower risk of developing insulin resistance or progressing from a prediabetic condition to diabetes.[6] According to the study, people who had the highest magnesium intake had only about half the risk (53 %) of developing compromised metabolic function or diabetes when compared with those who had the lowest magnesium intake. Acting promptly on this information can be life-changing for those who have been told by their physicians that their blood test results indicate that they are at a stage known as prediabetes.

Consider the popular Mediterranean Diet.

Why do you suppose the Mediterranean diet has been shown to be so effective for reducing the risk of heart disease, stroke, diabetes, and other health-related problems? Its effectiveness is probably due to the fact that the Mediterranean diet contains a relatively high level of magnesium (dailymail.co.uk,. updated 2016, December 8).[7] Likewise, there are various published studies that show that vegetarian or vegan diets in general typically provide similar health benefits. And of course, they too usually contain significantly higher levels of magnesium than the typical Western diet.

Magnesium deficiency appears to be the norm in today's world.

That suggests that any group that is able to avoid magnesium deficiency can be shown to have a lower risk of many of the most important health issues, including heart disease, stroke, and diabetes. King, Mainous, Geesey, & Woolson (2005) concluded that most Americans are magnesium deficient, and in addition, they proved that adequate magnesium intake lowers C-reactive protein (CRP) levels.[8] CRP is a measure of inflammation that has been shown to correlate with increased risk of cardiovascular disease.

Mazur et al. (2007) proved that only a few days of magnesium deficiency creates a condition of chronic inflammation in laboratory rats.[9] This inflammation syndrome involves leukocyte and macrophage activation, and the release of inflammatory cytokines along with other inflammatory agents. But when the researchers increased the magnesium in the cells of the rats, the inflammatory response was decreased. Mazur et al. (2007) pointed out that:

> *Moreover, magnesium deficiency induces a systemic stress response by activation of neuro endocrinological pathways. As nervous and immune systems interact bidirectionally, the roles of neuromediators have also been considered. Magesium [SIC] deficiency contributes to an exaggerated response to immune stress and oxidative stress is the consequence of the inflamma-*

What is Magnesium and Why Is It so Important?

tory response. Inflammation contributes to the pro-atherogenic changes in lipoprotein metabolism, endothelial dysfunction, thrombosis, hypertension and explains the aggravating effect of magnesium deficiency on the development of metabolic syndrome. (p. 48)

So we have published research that proves that a magnesium deficiency leads to an inflammatory state in the body, and this occurs independently of any other events. Since it's generally true that all autoimmune diseases are caused by chronic inflammation, this means that if we allow ourselves to become magnesium deficient, we are opening the door to the eventual development of one or more autoimmune diseases.

The particular autoimmune diseases that we may develop will be determines by our genes. And since autoimmune diseases like company, one autoimmune disease almost always leads to another. Knowing all this allows us to appreciate just how important magnesium is to our health, and helps us to understand why we need to be especially careful to avoid becoming magnesium deficient.

Chapter 2

Why Have so Many of Us Become Magnesium Deficient?

And why has the medical profession continued to ignore the problem?

Now why do you suppose most mainstream medical professionals seem to fail to appreciate the importance of magnesium? Apparently the problem is well entrenched within the medical profession. Here's an illustration of how ingrained that misguided attitude appears to be:

The University of Maryland Medical Center has a website that offers extensive information about magnesium (and many other topics).[10] If you look at the information listed there for magnesium, in their very first paragraph they claim:

Why Magnesium Is the Key to Long-Term Health

"Although you may not get enough magnesium from your diet, it is rare to be deficient in magnesium."

Really? Magnesium deficiency is rare? But we just got through looking at proof that not only is magnesium deficiency not rare, it's so common that the diets of a majority of Americans are magnesium deficient. The statement by the University of Maryland Medical Center appears to contradict itself. If we don't get an adequate amount of magnesium from our diet, where are they suggesting that we are supposed to get it? We're certainly not going to absorb magnesium from the air we breathe. At any rate, this misguided attitude clearly illustrates the naivety of mainstream medicine regarding magnesium. Magnesium is not even on their radar.

Roughly a quarter-century ago Ma et al. (1995) showed that magnesium deficiency is associated with numerous serious long-term health issues, including cardiovascular disease, hypertension, diabetes, insulin, and carotid arterial wall thickness.[11] The medical community seems to have lost touch with time-proven traditional methods in their endless pursuit of ever more powerful, increasingly-expensive drugs that only the rich can afford.

Why are so many people magnesium deficient?

It appears that our ancestors got most of their magnesium needs from the water they drank. Streams, rivers, and lakes previously contained high amounts of magnesium and other minerals that are important for health. Surface water running across soil and

Why Have so Many of Us Become Magnesium Deficient?

rocks that were once rich in magnesium and other minerals naturally absorbed significant amounts of many minerals. So our ancient ancestors didn't need any supplemental magnesium — they got plenty from their food and water.

In sharp contrast, these days water runs across soils and rocks that have been mostly depleted of magnesium by centuries of agricultural production. And to add insult to injury, those same soils and rocks have been contaminated by decades of chemical residue emissions and toxins from industrial plants and agricultural pesticides. And of course, in many cases the water itself has been directly contaminated.

Today, virtually all water distribution systems are filtered and otherwise treated to remove contaminants so that the water will be safe to drink, and in the process, almost all of the minerals that once were available in drinking water are removed. And to make doubly sure that all minerals are filtered out, these days many households use their own water filtration systems to obtain pure water. But pure water contains no minerals, so now our drinking water no longer supplies us with the minerals that were once available to our ancestors. So obviously we can no longer expect to get most of our magnesium from the water we drink.

Authorities point out that the average adult needs at least two liters of drinking water each day in order to maintain good health. In general, testing shows that in cities where water contains the highest amounts of magnesium, two liters of water contain only about 30 % of the recommended daily allowance

Why Magnesium Is the Key to Long-Term Health

(RDA) of magnesium Kiefer, 2007, February).[12] The same study found that in most cities, only about 10 to 20 % of the RDA for magnesium is available in two liters of water. But this is what's available in public water. By the time water goes through the additional purification equipment used in many homes, the amount of magnesium left in the water is virtually zero (history-ofwaterfilters.com, n.d.).[13]

Many people don't trust their water supply or for some other reason they drink bottled water. The purity of bottled water varies greatly, but other than a few European brands that are available in North America, both bottled and tap water in general contains very little magnesium (Azoulay, Garzon, & Eisenberg, 2001).[14]

Clearly, these days we must get the bulk of our magnesium needs from some other source. But this hasn't happened. Instead, we as a society have just ignored the increasing problem so that now most of us are magnesium deficient.

Why does the medical community continue to ignore this problem?

The fact that the medical community generally fails to recognize and address the growing problem with magnesium deficiency among the general public tends to amplify the problem. Part of the reason why physicians tend to overlook the problem is because the so-called "normal" range for an acceptable magnesium blood level may be too low (Liebscher & Liebscher, 2004).[15]

Why Have so Many of Us Become Magnesium Deficient?

The serum magnesium test is probably at the root of the problem.

The main reason why physicians fail to recognize the magnesium deficiency problem is that the serum magnesium test that is almost universally used by doctors to test a patient's magnesium level is only very weakly associated with the actual magnesium level of the cells of the body. The National Institutes of Health points out that less than one percent of the body's total supply of magnesium is available in blood serum. And since magnesium is a vital electrolyte, it's level is very closely regulated in the bloodstream within a rather narrow range.

That makes the serum test a very poor indicator of the actual magnesium level in the body. It's going to show a "normal" result unless an extreme condition is present. The body stores magnesium in the cells of the body whenever it is available, and then withdraws it as needed in order to keep the blood level of magnesium within a relatively narrow range. The serum magnesium test does not provide a way to read the amount of magnesium in the cells of the body. Therefore, a serum test cannot detect whether there is plenty of magnesium available in storage or whether the body will run out in a few hours (or a few minutes).

If you have ever been awakened by leg or foot cramps during the wee hours of the morning, that was probably caused by your body running low on magnesium, as it was pulling magnesium from your leg or foot muscles in order to keep the magnesium level of your blood from getting too low. Leg or foot cramps are most likely to occur during the night because this correlates with

Why Magnesium Is the Key to Long-Term Health

the length of time since the last meal that contained magnesium. It's an indication that you are magnesium deficient — you have inadequate magnesium reserves.

Obviously, this can lead to a dangerous situation since a severe magnesium deficiency can cause cardiac arrest. Surely, physicians are aware of this if they were awake during their anatomy classes, and yet they blithely continue to use the serum test, mostly because it's cheap, easy, and traditional to use. But because of their continued use of an inappropriate test, they are not even aware of the huge magnesium deficiency problem right under their noses.

And while the mainstream medical community continues to mostly ignore the problem, there is published medical research showing that simply correcting magnesium deficiencies could eliminate many serious health problems, including heart disease and hypertension (Touyz, 2004).[16] It could also eliminate many less serious, yet sometimes debilitating issues.

For example, many authorities believe that because of the fact that so many fibromyalgia patients are magnesium deficient, fibromyalgia may simply be a symptom of magnesium deficiency (Deans, 2012, September 11).[17] There is even published research showing that magnesium treats fibromyalgia (Engen et al., 2015).[18]

Why Have so Many of Us Become Magnesium Deficient?

Most people believe that they eat a healthy (nutritious) diet.
Many food shoppers carefully read labels on processed foods and make a serious effort to try to select foods so that they can provide a balanced diet for themselves and their families. The "health police" often assure us that following their recommendations will ensure good health for everyone. But out in the real world, it's pretty obvious that more and more people are developing allergies and food sensitivities and autoimmune diseases and cancer and various other health issues. Why isn't all the "expert" health advice working?

It's certainly possible that our food might not be as nutritious as we think it is?
Could some of the official RDA guidelines for vitamins and minerals be wrong? Is it possible that some of them might significantly understate optimal values for good health for many people? One of the serious problems with the RDA guidelines is that they assume that all people absorb nutrients at some arbitrary "normal" rate. RDA guidelines consider age, gender, pregnancy, and a few other categories. But out in the real world, even within those categories, not everyone absorbs nutrients at that so-called "normal" rate. The ability to absorb nutrients can vary widely, depending upon genetics, gut bacteria profiles, digestive health issues, disease, general health, exercise or physical activity levels, and possibly other conditions.

Numerous published research reports show that certain RDA listings are not consistent with current research. For example, compelling epidemiological evidence indicates that the RDA listings for vitamin D are only barely adequate for preventing the development of the disease known as rickets. For most people, much higher blood levels of vitamin D are necessary if they hope to prevent the development of most other diseases (Persky, 2013, pp. 87–88).[19] As soils become more and ,more depleted of magnesium and other minerals, are USDA published nutrient levels that were established decades ago, still accurate?

Consider some items in our diet that deplete magnesium?

Some of the foods that we eat or drink daily are known to deplete magnesium and possibly other nutrients, but it appears that issues such as these are totally ignored by the RDA guidelines. In order to obtain a one-size-fits-all number, the guidelines assume that everyone eats and drinks basically the same types of foods and that most forms of magnesium can be absorbed equally well. But that's a poor assumption because the various forms of magnesium vary widely in the rates at which they can be absorbed by the human digestive system. And some of us eat or drink substances that are known to deplete magnesium.

For example, coffee depletes magnesium.

And the more coffee one drinks, the greater the amount of magnesium that will be lost. Does the RDA for magnesium include an allowance for coffee? If it does, it is surely based on some arbitrary determination of the average amount of coffee in the American diet. Do you drink an "average" amount of coffee? If you drink more or less, then your magnesium needs will also

Why Have so Many of Us Become Magnesium Deficient?

be more or less, respectively. But it's very likely that the RDA doesn't have a builtin allowance for coffee, so anyone who drinks coffee is likely to gradually become magnesium deficient, even if they follow RDA guidelines. And higher than normal coffee consumption will lead to an even more significant magnesium deficiency. Alcohol is also known to deplete magnesium. Other foods such as tea, carbonated drinks, sugar and sweet foods in general, are also known to deplete magnesium.

Many medications deplete magnesium.

The list includes various types of medications, including corticosteroids, certain antibiotics, antacids, contraceptives, cardiovascular medications. diuretics, proton pump inhibitors (PPIs), and possibly others. Such medications don't necessarily totally prevent the absorption of magnesium, and their effects may vary from one individual to the next, but for most people, they can reduce the absorption of magnesium enough to cause a significant reduction in cellular magnesium levels.

As an example of how extensively some drugs can interfere with the absorption of magnesium, consider the first paragraph of a warning issued by the FDA regarding the use of proton pump inhibitors (FDA Drug Safety Communication, 2011, March 2):[20]

> *[3-2-2011] The U.S. Food and Drug Administration (FDA) is informing the public that prescription proton pump inhibitor (PPI) drugs may cause low serum magnesium levels (hypomagnesemia) if taken for prolonged periods of time (in most cases, longer than one year).* ***In approximately one-quarter of the cases reviewed, magnesium supplementation alone***

> *did not improve low serum magnesium levels and the PPI had to be discontinued.*

Note the last sentence in the quote, which I have emphasized with bold print. This is a very, very serious health issue, to say the least.

Our paleolithic ancestors didn't drink coffee or alcohol, nor did they use medications.

It's certainly possible that they may have used a variety of natural remedies for various health issues, but it's not likely that they used any treatments that depleted magnesium. Consequently our digestive system evolved without any allowance for magnesium-depleting foods, beverages, or medications.

Our great-grandparents used far fewer magnesium-depleting drugs than the generations that have come after them. And the parents of our great-grandparents used even fewer magnesium-depleting substances. The problem of depleting magnesium has increased exponentially in the last few decades and it appears that the lion's share of the blame may go to our increasing use of magnesium-wasting medications.

But our magnesium deficiency problem cannot be blamed on any one cause. With a combination of declining magnesium availability in agricultural soils, improved water filtration and treatment methods, diets that sometimes deplete magnesium,

Why Have so Many of Us Become Magnesium Deficient?

and the increasing use of magnesium-depleting drugs, it's no wonder that most of us are magnesium deficient.

Chapter 3

How Accurate Are the Magnesium Tests Used by Doctors?

And how can I tell if I'm magnesium deficient?

We've already discussed why the magnesium test most often ordered by doctors fails to reliably measure our body's actual magnesium level. Here's part of what the National Institutes of Health says about magnesium. Take note of the last sentence in the quote, which I have emphasized with red print:

> *An adult body contains approximately 25 g magnesium, with 50% to 60% present in the bones and most of the rest in soft tissues. Less than 1% of total magnesium is in blood serum, and these levels are kept under tight control. Normal serum magnesium concentrations range between 0.75 and 0.95*

millimoles (mmol)/L. Hypomagnesemia is defined as a serum magnesium level less than 0.75 mmol/L. Magnesium homeostasis is largely controlled by the kidney, which typically excretes about 120 mg magnesium into the urine each day. Urinary excretion is reduced when magnesium status is low.

Assessing magnesium status is difficult because most magnesium is inside cells or in bone. The most commonly used and readily available method for assessing magnesium status is measurement of serum magnesium concentration, even though serum levels have little correlation with total body magnesium levels or concentrations in specific tissues.

The red blood cell (RBC) test is not perfect, but it's much, much better than the serum test for measuring magnesium levels.

This is still a blood test, but it measures the amount of magnesium in our red blood cells, and this is representative of the amount of magnesium available in other cells in the body. The main problem with the serum test is that if we have recently eaten a meal that contains magnesium, or taken a magnesium supplement, a serum magnesium test is always going to show a normal level. But if we have virtually no reserves, as soon as the magnesium currently in our blood is used up, our blood level of magnesium is going to drop drastically, (because we have no reserves to draw from). In extreme cases, this might happen a few hours, or even a few minutes after the blood draw. The proper place for the serum magnesium test is in the emergency room, where medical professionals need to evaluate a patient's

How Accurate Are the Magnesium Tests Used by Doctors?

current status, and have no interest in reserves. For any other purpose, the RBC magnesium test is far superior to the serum test. For the record, a couple of much more accurate magnesium tests have been developed, but they are rarely used.

A test known as the ionized magnesium test is more accurate, but sadly, it's only available at a few select locations. The Energy Dispersive X-Ray Analysis (EXA) test is the most accurate magnesium test of all. It's based on the analysis of tissue samples scraped from the inside of the patient's cheeks. But similar to the ionized magnesium test, locating a doctor or a lab that's set up to do this test can be a challenge. So our best bet is the RBC magnesium test.

Dr. Carolyn Dean is a magnesium expert who has written several books about magnesium and she even has her own line of magnesium supplements that are more easily absorbed than conventional magnesium supplements. She claims that the so-called "normal range" of test results for even the RBC magnesium test is inaccurate because it was developed using results from a group of subjects 80 % of whom were magnesium deficient. She points out that this skewed the results toward the low side, and she insists that the actual normal range should be higher. In her opinion, the normal range for the RBC test should be 6.0–6.5 ng/ml (15–16.2 nmol/l) rather than the wider and usually lower range used by most laboratories (Dean, C., 2015, October 20).[21]

Why Magnesium Is the Key to Long-Term Health

Do you crave chocolate?
Chocolate contains a significant amount of magnesium. Medical statistics show that people who are magnesium deficient often crave chocolate.

Leg or foot cramps are usually due to magnesium deficiency and they're easily eliminated by magnesium.
Restless leg syndrome is another problem that magnesium resolves. These symptoms are usually caused by a magnesium deficiency and magnesium usually resolves them. A deficiency of other electrolytes (such as potassium, calcium, or sodium) can also cause leg or foot cramps, but magnesium deficiency seems to be the most common electrolyte deficiency by far.

Brittle nails are another indication of a long-term magnesium deficiency.
Many people mistakenly believe that a calcium deficiency is the cause of brittle nails, but this is not the case. Magnesium and vitamin D regulate calcium utilization. Almost everyone has sufficient calcium in their diet. So when issues that appear to be associated with a calcium deficiency show up (such as osteoporosis, for example), it's time to suspect either a vitamin D or a magnesium deficiency, or both. A chronic magnesium deficiency can definitely cause brittle nails, and a moderate to severe deficiency can cause slow nail growth.

How Accurate Are the Magnesium Tests Used by Doctors?

In some cases there can be many other symptoms of magnesium deficiency.

Of course not everyone who is magnesium deficient will have all of these symptoms, and some symptoms may go unnoticed or they may be attributed to some other cause, but all of the symptoms listed here are known to be associated with magnesium deficiency. And in most cases, taking an adequate magnesium supplement will resolve these symptoms.

Magnesium deficiency symptoms can also include (but are not limited to) muscle weakness, muscle twitches, pain, tremors, tingling or numbness in hands or feet, low energy, fatigue, unexplained weight loss, insomnia, heart palpitations or tachycardia (high heart rate), irritability , profuse sweating, shortness of breath or the inability to draw a deep breath, hypertension or erratic blood pressure, migraines, recurring skin or urinary tract infections, recurring vaginal yeast infections, brain fog, depression, constipation, foul body odor, frequent urination, urination urgency, kidney stones, kidney disease, dry mouth, excessive thirst, dry itchy skin, tooth decay, osteoporosis, confusion, irritability, anxiety, panic attacks, apathy, anorexia, memory problems, and compromised learning ability (University of Maryland Medical Center, n.d., Sircus, 2009, December 8, Schachter, 1996).[22,23,24] Please note that some of these symptoms are the same symptoms that are often seen with diabetes because (as we discussed in chapter 1) magnesium deficiency causes insulin resistance and reduced insulin production by the pancreas.

Why Magnesium Is the Key to Long-Term Health

Few people associate a magnesium deficiency with nausea.

But believe it or not, a persistent nausea problem is sometimes just a symptom of a chronic magnesium deficiency. One of the most well-known examples of persistent nausea is the "morning sickness" that often develops during the first trimester of pregnancy. It's traditionally blamed on the hormonal changes that occur during pregnancy. And this is partially correct. But as is usually the case, the devil is in the details. What actually happens is that the escalating estrogen levels deplete the mother-to-be's reserve supply of magnesium (Dean, 2011, February 20).[25] Remember that constipation is a symptom of magnesium deficiency, so this also explains the constipation that's so common with pregnancy.

This happens because as the fetus begins to develop, a huge boost in the demand for magnesium occurs in order to build healthy bones and supply all the other magnesium-based needs for both the mother and fetus. Unless supplemental magnesium is supplied, a magnesium deficiency often develops within a few weeks. So it's actually the magnesium deficiency that causes the nausea described as "morning sickness". Women who build up adequate magnesium reserves early on in the process can prevent or minimize morning sickness and various other problems (Zarean & Tarjan, 2017).[26] Clearly, magnesium deficiency can cause nausea.

How Accurate Are the Magnesium Tests Used by Doctors?

Do you often feel as though you need to take a deep breath — but you can't?

This is a symptom of chronic magnesium deficiency that's not often discussed and it's virtually never on doctors' radar. Breathing is normally automatically controlled by the autonomic nervous system. A chronic magnesium deficiency can interfere with the proper functioning of smooth muscle tissue by causing it to spasm, including the diaphragm that allows us to breathe. When a breathing issue occurs because of an acute magnesium deficiency, the patient will become very aware of her or his breathing. Almost every breath will become a conscious effort, and there will be an urgent desire to take a deep breath. But most attempts will not be productive. These episodes often occur late at night, and sometimes the patient will wonder if she or he woke up because their body forgot to breathe, and they will be afraid to go back to sleep for fear of not awakening the next time it happens. This leads to anxiety, another common but seldom-recognized symptom of magnesium deficiency.

Breathing can even seem labored, almost like an asthma attack except that there will be no wheezing. When patients ask their doctors for an explanation of what might be causing such symptoms, the response will probably be a blank stare, because physicians are typically not properly trained to recognize magnesium deficiency symptoms, so they are not likely to be familiar with this problem. When they listen to the patient's breathing through their stethoscope, it will sound normal, so they will conclude that there's nothing wrong — therefore the problem must be due to the patient's imagination.

Why Magnesium Is the Key to Long-Term Health

If you're wondering how I am able to describe this issue in such detail — I've been there. I've experienced everything described here and I can assure you that when it happens in the middle of the night especially, it grabs your attention. It's a very frustrating symptom. I can also assure you that taking an adequate magnesium supplement will completely resolve this issue.

In some situations, doctors will diagnose this condition as hyperventilation disorder (if they diagnose anything at all). But the root cause is a chronic magnesium deficiency. The issue appears to be associated with compromised nerve function and weakened muscle response by the diaphragm, which results in reduced breathing capacity. This observation is supported by research that shows that children who are magnesium deficient often have reduced lung function (Gilliland, Berhane, Li, Kim, & Margolis, 2002).[27] But apparently this isn't a part of medical school training, so if patients who have this problem don't figure out what's causing it themselves, it may never be resolved.

Sometimes magnesium deficiency can cause seizures.

Case studies suggest that in some situations a chronic magnesium deficiency can eventually lead to epileptic seizures (Nuytten, Van Hees, Meulemans, & Carton, 1991).[28] In addition, there are published research studies showing that in general, people who have epilepsy tend to have lower magnesium levels than people who do not have the condition (Yuen, & Sander, 2012).[29] Whether magnesium deficiency might play a role in causing epilepsy or epilepsy depletes magnesium, remains to be seen, but some researchers have suggested that magnesium

How Accurate Are the Magnesium Tests Used by Doctors?

supplementation might be successfully used to reduce epileptic seizures.

In some cases, magnesium deficiency may be caused by genetics.

According to research, some people are unable to absorb magnesium as well as others because of their genetics (Mauskop, & Varughese, 2012).[30] Various other issues can either compromise the absorption of magnesium or cause it to be wasted by the renal system. Galland (1991–1992) pointed out, that even psychological stress can cause magnesium to be wasted by the kidneys, resulting in a magnesium deficiency.[31]

Are you depressed?

There's evidence that many (if not most) cases of depression may be due to magnesium deficiency. Eby & Eby (2006) published case studies showing that supplementing with magnesium often brings rapid resolution of depression symptoms, (in addition to resolving many other health issues).[32] It's not likely that any significant research using magnesium as a treatment for depression will be done in the future, however, because most research is financed by the big pharmaceutical companies. Big Pharma is making far too much money from the sale of over-priced medications to treat anxiety and depression for them to consider jeopardizing sales by proving that something as cheap as magnesium is just as effective. That would be counterproductive, so it's not going to happen.

Chapter 4

What Types of Magnesium Are Available for Supplementing?

Why some magnesium supplements are much better than others

Magnesium for use as a supplement is always available as a compound with some other element, never in the pure state. That may seem counterproductive, but this is done for a very good reason — pure magnesium powder is very explosive. So it has to be stabilized by combining it with another element to eliminate the risk of explosion. Depending on the nature of the combination, the specific magnesium compounds have varying degrees of absorbability, percentages of magnesium, and different pharmaceutical characteristics.

How we take magnesium supplements can affect how well we absorb them.

If we take large doses of magnesium at one time, this can result in wasted magnesium. As the blood level of magnesium increases, the absorption rate tends to decline. So if we divide the total daily dose into several smaller amounts and take them at various times during the day, (preferably at mealtimes), we will be able to absorb magnesium more efficiently. Magnesium supplements typically work best when taken with a meal, but taking them with food is not mandatory.

Various magnesium compounds have different rates of absorption

Magnesium is available in many different forms and some forms are much easier to absorb than others. Any magnesium that is not absorbed will remain in the intestines (along with other waste material), and if the amount of magnesium supplement that is swallowed is large enough, and if enough of it is not absorbed, the unabsorbed magnesium that remains in the intestines may act as a laxative.

Quite a few types of magnesium supplements are available.

Choosing the right type can make the difference between resolving a deficiency and just causing diarrhea. Commonly-available magnesium compounds include (but are not limited to) these forms:

What Types of Magnesium Are Available for Supplementing?

magnesium oxide
magnesium chloride
magnesium sulfate
magnesium carbonate
chelated magnesium (magnesium glycinate)
magnesium orotate
magnesium citrate
magnesium maleate
magnesium gluconate
magnesium threonate

These compounds contain different amounts of magnesium, and the magnesium contained in the various types tends to have differing rates at which it can be absorbed by the human digestive system. For example, for lotions and oils and other products designed to be absorbed through the skin, Ancient Minerals shows these amounts of elemental magnesium for their products (Ashley, 2012, February 10).[33]

magnesium Oil: 560mg per teaspoon*
magnesium Gel: 490mg per teaspoon
magnesium Bath Flakes: 15g per cup
magnesium Lotion: 185mg per teaspoon

*8 sprays of Magnesium Oil equals roughly 100mg of magnesium.

Magnesium oxide.
The cheapest and most dense form of magnesium is magnesium oxide. Because it's cheap, it's naturally the type most commonly

found in mineral supplements and multivitamins. It's also the type most commonly used by hospitals. Magnesium oxide contains 300 mg of elemental magnesium per 500 mg tablet (which is a high percentage, and makes magnesium oxide the densest form of magnesium supplements available). But it has the poorest absorption rate of all the common forms of magnesium. Human digestive systems can only absorb up to about 4 % of the magnesium in magnesium oxide. The rest stays in the intestines where it tends to mix with water and form magnesium hydroxide, otherwise known as milk of magnesia, a common laxative. That characteristic makes magnesium oxide a rather poor choice as a magnesium supplement.

Magnesium chloride.

Since magnesium chloride is soluble in water (this is the form found in sea water) it's often available as a liquid intended to be sprayed or wiped onto the skin. It can also be used in a bath or a foot soak. Magnesium chloride contains about 25 % elemental magnesium, but when dissolved in water, the amount of magnesium available depends on the dilution.

When applying it to the skin, some people leave magnesium oil or lotion in place after it soaks in, while others prefer to apply it 20 or 30 minutes before taking a bath or shower. For spray products, it's usually best to spray it into the palm of one's hand and then rub it on the skin because any spray that misses the mark and lands on the floor can create slick spots that might cause someone to slip and fall.

What Types of Magnesium Are Available for Supplementing?

Magnesium sulfate.

Magnesium sulfate is another form that's water soluble. The popular product Epsom Salt belongs to this category. Similar to magnesium chloride, the amount of magnesium available in a solution of magnesium sulfate depends on the dilution.

Magnesium chloride and magnesium sulfate are the forms usually chosen for topical applications. The former is usually used for oils and lotions, while the latter is usually chosen for foot soaks and for adding to bathwater. In cases where digestive system sensitivity is so high that oral magnesium supplements are not well-tolerated, topical applications of magnesium may be a better choice. Some people prefer to use a combination of oral magnesium and topical applications in order to be able to absorb an adequate amount of magnesium without upsetting their digestive system.

Magnesium carbonate.

Magnesium carbonate contains about 125 mg of elemental magnesium per 500 mg tablet. Compared with the other forms, it's relatively poorly absorbed.

Magnesium glycinate.

Chelated magnesium (magnesium glycinate) is magnesium bound to the amino acids glycine and lysine. Because amino acids are readily absorbed, magnesium glycinate is well-absorbed and very bioavailable. It usually contains 100 mg of elemental magnesium in each tablet. Magnesium glycinate is one of the more expensive forms of magnesium, but this form of magnesium is one of the least-likely to cause diarrhea when larger doses are used. For most people, this is typically a good choice for a magnesium supplement.

Beware of products sold as "Buffered Chelated Magnesium" because in many cases the buffering agent appears to be cheap magnesium oxide. Such products may have as much as 50 % of the chelated magnesium replaced with magnesium oxide, making Buffered Chelated Magnesium a rather poor choice as a magnesium supplement for most people.

Magnesium orotate.
Magnesium orotate only contains 31 mg of elemental magnesium per 500 mg tablet. So the amount of magnesium supplied is rather minimal, but it's normally well-absorbed.

Magnesium citrate.
Magnesium citrate contains 80 mg of elemental magnesium in each 500 mg tablet. It's usually well-absorbed, and works well as a magnesium supplement as long as the dose is small to moderate (such as at or below the RDA). Higher doses may act as a laxative, but individual tolerances can vary.

Magnesium maleate.
Magnesium maleate is not as commonly-used as some of the other forms. It contains 56 mg of elemental magnesium, which makes it one of the less-potent forms of magnesium.

What Types of Magnesium Are Available for Supplementing?

Magnesium gluconate.
Magnesium gluconate contains 27 mg of elemental magnesium per 500 mg tablet, making it a rather weak magnesium supplement. But it's easily absorbed, and rated as relatively quick-acting.

Be sure to read both front and back labels carefully.
Reading the labels carefully when selecting a dose of oral magnesium is important, because magnesium labels can sometimes be misleading. Some manufacturers show the amount of magnesium on the front label as the "serving size" rather than the amount of magnesium in each tablet. The back label then specifies how many tablets comprise the "serving size". This type of labeling can be confusing, and it's easy to end up taking half as much magnesium as you intended. So be sure that you read and understand both the front and back labels carefully.

What about magnesium threonate?
Magnesium threonate (magnesium L-threonate) is not a conventional magnesium supplement. Research shows that it can cross the blood/brain barrier to affect pain perception in the brain. Previous clinical studies have shown that chronic pain causes short-term memory (STM) deficits in approximately two-thirds of patients. Wang et al., (2013) showed (on an animal model) that magnesium L-threonate is capable of preventing and restoring short term memory deficits due to chronic neuropathic pain.[34]

Why Magnesium Is the Key to Long-Term Health

Magnesium threonate is currently being promoted as the ultimate form of magnesium. It's claimed to stop brain aging, memory loss, and various other things, but one thing to keep in mind is that to date, only animal studies have been published. No medically-approved studies have been done on humans. Until such data from studies on human subjects have been published, all the hype is strictly speculation. So if you are considering using magnesium threonate, proceed with caution. And keep in mind that this is still an experimental drug, rather than a proven medication.

Chapter 5

What Else Should We Know About Magnesium?

What else can magnesium do for us?

How is magnesium absorbed by the digestive system?

Normally, we absorb about 11 % of our magnesium in the duodenum (the first segment of the small intestine) and we absorb about 22 % in the jejunum, which is the second segment of the small intestine, (Albion Laboratories, Inc., n.d.).[35] About 56 % is absorbed in the ileum (the last segment of the small intestine) and the other 11 % is absorbed in the colon (Albion Laboratories, Inc., n.d.). Both the ileum and the colon are usually inflamed in the case of most microscopic colitis patients and many Crohn's patients, for example (Koskela, 2011, DiLauro & Crum-Cianflone, 2010)[36, 37].

So it shouldn't be surprising that IBDs tend to severely deplete magnesium.

Because fully two-thirds of magnesium absorption takes place in inflamed segments of the intestine (and we know that inflammation limits the absorption of nutrients), it's almost inevitable that IBD patients will become progressively magnesium deficient.

Adequate magnesium is necessary for proper immune system functioning.

Because of this, magnesium deficiency may be implicated in most or all autoimmune syndromes. Consider that Cojocaru, Cojocaru, Tănăsescu, Iacob, & Iliescu, (2009). found that during and after episodes of major bacterial infections, serum (blood) levels of magnesium decrease significantly within a few days of the onset and this continues for several weeks.[38] This indicates that magnesium is being used at a much higher rate than normal when the immune system is fighting a bacterial infection

Most inflammatory bowel diseases (IBDs) except for celiac disease have long been suspected to be caused by bacterial infections or adverse gut biome changes. Perhaps this is another reason why all IBDs tend to deplete magnesium.

The leading cause of hypothyroidism in the U.S.A. is Hashimoto's disease.

Hashimoto's is one of the common autoimmune diseases. Magnesium is known to be very important for the activation of thyroid hormone T4 (Kent, 2015, November 11).[39] Without suffi-

What Else Should We Know About Magnesium?

cient magnesium, T4 cannot be activated into the usable form, T3. Someone who has a magnesium deficiency will not be able to resolve their hypothyroidism symptoms, even if they are taking a T4 supplement such as levothyroxine sodium (Synthroid). Their body will not be able to convert the T4 into T3, so they will remain short of T3.

Many physicians tend to refuse to issue a prescription for a natural desiccated thyroid hormone product (which contains T3) in order to address this problem, because they don't understand that magnesium is required to make the conversion. Consequently they mistakenly insist that synthetic T4 should be a sufficient treatment. And of course they also fail to prescribe magnesium, so there are many hypothyroid patients for whom their prescribed thyroid hormone treatment does not work to relieve their symptoms.

If you are magnesium-deficient, you might also be iron-deficient.

This often happens because the same foods often contain both magnesium and iron, so if your diet is short of one, there is a good chance that it may be short of the other. And the absorption of magnesium together with iron seems to be synergistic.

That is, when they both are ingested together, this seems to result in better absorption rates for both than when they are ingested separately. But the point is that if you are magnesium deficient, you are probably also iron-deficient. Conversely. if you have anemia, you almost surely have a magnesium deficiency also.

Correcting a magnesium deficiency is almost always much easier to do than correcting an iron deficiency. Most iron supplements are hard on the stomach, so most people have to use them in moderation. Blackstrap molasses seems to work about as well as anything, but it usually takes a long time to resolve an iron deficiency.

Many popular beverages contain high amounts of phosphorous.

Too much phosphorous in one's diet can interfere with the absorption of magnesium, iron, and calcium (Keefer, 2017, October 3).).[40] Fruit juices such as orange juice, apple juice, grape juice, and many others, and carbonated beverages such as sodas, mineral waters, seltzers, and many sports drinks contain relatively high levels of phosphorous.

Too much calcium in the diet can cause an iron deficiency.

Calcium is the only substance that is known to be capable of inhibiting both the heme and non-heme forms of iron. But there are other foods such as cocoa, tea, and coffee that can interfere with the absorption of one or the other forms of iron.

Do you have allergy symptoms?

Histamine is an organic nitrogen compound that's normally released by the immune system in response to either or both local and systemic immune system stimulations. Consequently, it can have both local and systemic effects. Histamine is released

What Else Should We Know About Magnesium?

by mast cells, and by white cells such as basophils or eosinophils. It's used by the immune system to modulate subsequent responses. As a messenger, histamine can act both as a physiological function regulator, and a neurotransmitter.

Histamine is responsible for most of the classic allergy symptoms when we experience a pollen allergy or some other type of common allergy reaction. The runny nose, watery eyes, itching, and in more severe reactions, the anaphylactic symptoms such as airway restriction and breathing difficulties are all due to the release of large amounts of histamine. When we get bit by a mosquito or stung by a wasp, the redness and swelling that develops is due to the release of histamine in the tissues surrounding the bite or sting.

Histamine causes increased permeability (porosity) of the small blood vessels (capillaries) in the area so that the immune system can pass white blood cells from the capillaries into the surrounding tissues to confront any pathogens or toxins that might be present. This causes the redness, swelling, and general inflammation as the histamine and white cells, and fluids from the bloodstream flow into the area.

Histamine is derived from histidine, an essential amino acid, in the body. Because we cannot produce histidine, it must be available in the diet. However, certain species of gut bacteria are capable of producing histidine, so it's possible for an imbalance of gut bacteria (dysbiosis) to cause an imbalance that might affect our immune system and cause it to produce excess histamine.

While normal amounts of histamine are necessary for the proper functioning of certain digestive processes (for example, when we smell food, histamine is released in the stomach to trigger the release of gastric acid to prepare for an expected meal), an excessive amount can produce various types of undesirable effects.

Histamine issues are associated with a magnesium deficiency.

Over three decades ago, Nishio, Ishiguro, & Miyao proved that rats fed a magnesium-deficient diet showed significantly increased histamine levels in their urine after four days, and the histamine levels peaked out on the eighth day.[41] The rat's tissues also showed an increase in histamine levels by the eighth day. When the magnesium-deficient rats were fed a diet containing a higher amount of magnesium for two days, their histamine and serum magnesium levels returned to the same levels as the controls in the study. So clearly, a magnesium deficiency can cause elevated histamine levels.

Could Parkinson's and Alzheimer's disease be symptoms of a chronic magnesium deficiency?

The Michael J Fox Foundation, points out that almost 80 % of Parkinson's patients have constipation. And the constipation usually begins several years before the Parkinson's symptoms begin to show up (Dolhun, 2014, December 08).[42] As we have already seen in previous discussions in this book, constipation is a very common symptom of magnesium deficiency

What Else Should We Know About Magnesium?

Furthermore, the Michael J Fox Foundation also points out that a certain protein that's found in clumps in the brains of all Parkinson's disease patients can also be found in certain other locations in the body outside of the brain, including the enteric nervous system. This protein is known as alpha-synuclein). The enteric nervous system is made up of the nerves that control the digestive system, and it's sometimes referred to as the second brain (Dolhun, 2014, December 08). The question of interest here is whether alpha-synuclein might develop in the gut first, and then spread to the brain where it eventually causes motor symptoms.

We know from published research that Parkinson's patients have lower vitamin D levels than people who don't have Parkinson's, (Kwon et al., 2016).[43] We also know magnesium has been shown to prevent the clumping of alpha-synuclein (Golts et al., 2002).[44] That suggests that a chronic magnesium deficiency might allow a buildup of clumps of alpha-synuclein.

A similar situation exists with Alzheimer's disease, with neurofibrillary tangles known as tau in the brain of Alzheimer's patients (Guo et al., 2013).[45] So far no one has published proof that magnesium resolves neurofibrillary tangles, but some neurologists have already begun experimenting with using magnesium to treat Alzheimer's patients (Jones, 2013, May 27).[46] My point here is that Alzheimer's and Parkinson's diseases may not actually be diseases so much as they might be symptoms of decades of ignoring a magnesium deficiency.

Remember — vitamin D and magnesium work together to protect the immune system and keep it working properly. We discussed on page two of chapter one that adequate magnesium is necessary in order to activate vitamin D so that the immune system can use it to defend the body against all types of adverse events. Perhaps some form of magnesium threonate may eventually be shown to be advantageous for treating or preventing neurodegenerative diseases such as Alzheimer's and Parkinson's disease.

A sudden magnesium deficiency (rather than hormonal changes) causes common PMS symptoms.

True, hormonal changes such as increasing estrogen and progesterone levels during the second half of the menstrual cycle are the cause of a dramatic magnesium level decline, but it's the resulting magnesium deficiency that actually causes the symptoms (Fischer, 2017, September 21).[47] The large magnesium level decline can cause spasms in the arteries that supply blood to the brain — the result is PMS symptoms and migraines. The symptoms can be reduced by significantly boosting magnesium reserves (by taking additional supplemental magnesium) before the symptoms develop. It's very common to crave chocolate before menses. This happens because dark chocolate (with at least 80 % cocoa content) contains more magnesium than any other type of food.

What Else Should We Know About Magnesium?

Research shows that taking a full RDA of magnesium cuts the risk of developing pancreatic cancer in half.

In 2015, Dibaba, Xun, Yokota, White, and He published a very interesting study based on data collected between the years of 2000–2008, concerning the use of magnesium supplements.[48] The study involved 66,806 men and women aged 50–76 years (when the study began). The subjects were ranked according to the percentage of magnesium supplements that they used, relative to the recommended daily allowance (RDA).

The National Institutes of Health recommends that men in this age range need an RDA of 420 mg of magnesium and women need 320 mg (Magnesium Fact Sheet for Health Professionals, 2016, February 11).[49] Of course the RDA includes all sources of magnesium in someone's diet, whether from food alone or food plus a supplement. This particular study ignored all of the magnesium in all of the subject's food. It considered only supplemental magnesium..

With that in mind, this particular study showed that compared with those who took the full RDA, those who took from 75–99 % of the RDA had a 42 % increased risk of developing pancreatic cancer. It showed that those who took less than 75 % of the RDA had a 76 % increased risk of developing pancreatic cancer. Obviously, for a study involving such a large number of subjects, these results indicate a very strong correlation.

Why Magnesium Is the Key to Long-Term Health

These study results tell us that taking a full RDA of magnesium cuts the risk of pancreatic cancer approximately in half. Remember, this isn't just a projection — it's what actually happened to the people in this study. And also remember that this study only considered the amount of supplemental magnesium taken by the subjects.

Now let's look at a real-life example of how a chronic magnesium deficiency may have initiated a life-changing event.

Let's use the information we've learned to reanalyze a very famous case of pancreatic cancer — Steve Jobs' case. Steve Jobs had an uncommon form of pancreatic cancer (PC) known as a neuroendocrine tumor. About 5 % of PC cases involve this type of cancer which grows and spreads much more slowly than the more common form known as pancreatic adenocarcinoma (Gardner, n.d.).[50] Neuroendocrine tumors develop in islet cells in the pancreas. These cells produce hormones to regulate certain body functions.

Pancreatic adenocarcinomas develop in the ductal cells that line the drainage tubes of the pancreas, and as previously mentioned, they tend to be far more aggressive than the neuroendocrine tumors. Pancreatic adenocarcinomas are the type that are usually referred to as simply "pancreatic cancer". Because Steve Jobs had the less-aggressive neuroendocrine type, he was able to survive for eight years after it was diagnosed in 2003.

What Else Should We Know About Magnesium?

Apparently (due to the fact that it was slow-growing) the cancer had existed for many years before it was diagnosed. And his surgery in 2004 revealed that the cancer had existed for so long that it had spread to his liver. Growth rates for this type of cancer are relatively well established. Using the diameter of the liver tumor and working backward to calculate the growth rate of the cancer, Dr. John McDougal extrapolated that the cancer had probably spread to the liver about seven years earlier (McDougall, 2011, November).[51]

That suggests that Jobs had lived with the cancer at least 15 years after it had spread to his liver. That implies that the original pancreatic cancer would likely have had to begin at least several years prior to that (because cancers typically do not metastasize until they have developed for at least several years).

Looking at other information from his past, consider a report that indicated that in 1987 his hands had a yellow appearance. Jaundice is a well-known side effect in some cases of pancreatic cancer. This suggests that the cancer had already existed 24 years before his death. Dr. McDougal used this and other information to estimate that the pancreatic cancer may have originated when Jobs was in his early to mid-twenties. This would have been approximately 30 years before his death.

This suggests that Steve Jobs' vegan and sometimes fruitarian diet might have slowed down the growth of the tumor. But the problem with that observation is the fact that his diet may have also helped create an ideal environment for the development of pancreatic cancer.

Pancreatic cancer uses fructose to rapidly divide and grow new cells.

Vegan diets, and especially fruitarian diets, contain high amounts of the sugar fructose. While it's true that most types of cancer cells tend to thrive on sugar of any type, researchers (Liu et al., 2010) showed that because of the unique way that fructose is metabolized in the body, pancreatic cancer cells are able to exploit fructose to supercharge their reproductive ability (Liu et al., 2010).[52] Unlike other sugars, fructose is metabolized in the liver. That means that no insulin response is generated (Ancira, updated 2018, April 06).[53] Liu et al. (2010) made this important observation:

> These findings show that cancer cells can readily metabolize fructose to increase proliferation. They have major significance for cancer patients given dietary refined fructose consumption, and indicate that efforts to reduce refined fructose intake or inhibit fructose-mediated actions may disrupt cancer growth. (p. 6,368)

Steve Jobs body odor problem is another powerful clue.

Here's why this suggests that he had a chronic magnesium deficiency beginning at an early age. His body odor problem was well-documented (Mertz, 2014).[54] It's obvious that most people have just assumed that this problem was due to Jobs not bathing often enough. And it is true that after he adopted a fruit and vegetable diet he decided that his diet would make him immune to body odor so he decided to stop bathing regularly. But it's not

What Else Should We Know About Magnesium?

clear that failure to bathe often enough was the initial cause of his body odor when he was younger. I can use my own experience with magnesium deficiency to shed some light on this situation.

In 2015 I had a severe magnesium deficiency brought on by a series of three back-to-back antibiotic treatments for dental work that depleted what was left of my meager magnesium reserves. I apparently already had a chronic magnesium deficiency due to a restricted diet because of food sensitivities). I can tell you that a major magnesium deficiency can cause one's body odor to become not just unpleasant, but downright putrid. I couldn't believe it — to put it bluntly, I smelled badly enough to knock a buzzard off a perch above a dead carcass over a quarter-mile away. Taking a shower every night helped, but that didn't resolve the problem.

I was so low on magnesium that I had a very severe reaction. I would wake up in the wee hours of the morning, sweating profusely (even though the room was very cool). My heart rate would be over a hundred and my blood pressure would be very low. My breathing would was shallow and rapid. And amazingly, not one of my doctors ever connected my symptoms with magnesium deficiency.

Finally, my symptoms became so bad that I couldn't force myself to eat breakfast one morning, so I went to the Emergency Room (ER). One of the blood tests they did was a serum magnesium test. After the doctor reviewed the test results, he informed me that "everything looked fine" on the tests, so they sent me home with no treatment. Fortunately, I reviewed the test results the following day and I noticed that the magnesium test result was flagged as low. I was already taking 300 mg of magnesium daily, so I doubled my dose. The next day I was fine — all of my symptoms were gone, including the obnoxious body odor.

Now obviously, Steve Jobs' magnesium deficiency was not as severe as mine, but it was almost surely the initial reason for his obnoxious body odor. Magnesium deficiency is not even on most doctors' radar. So if Steve Jobs had a magnesium deficiency, there is no way in the world that any of them would have ever detected it. Obviously, this is an important clue, because as we discussed a few pages ago, a magnesium deficiency significantly increases the risk of developing pancreatic cancer.

Another clue can be found in the fact that he often had problems with kidney stones.

Kidney stones can be a symptom of magnesium deficiency. Again, I can verify this by personal experience, as I had the same problem as my magnesium deficiency became worse. In fact, the only kidney stones I ever had in my life sent me to the Emergency Room about six months before my increasing magnesium deficiency symptoms became severe enough to cause me to make that visit to the ER described on the previous page.

Kidney problems apparently were the reason why Jobs had scheduled the scan in 2003 that revealed the spot on his pancreas and lead to his diagnosis of pancreatic cancer. But he had been dealing with kidney issues for years. So we have plenty of reasons to suspect that he may have been magnesium deficient

What Else Should We Know About Magnesium?

for many years. The problem probably went all the way back to his childhood. As we saw back in chapter 3 on page 29, some people are magnesium deficient because of genetics (Mauskop, & Varughese, 2012).

Looking at all the evidence, there's no justification to claim that magnesium deficiency was the cause of his cancer, although it might have increased his risk. He was probably just a victim of misfortune.

But what is absolutely amazing here is that despite his celebrity, and the fact that he interacted with many people (and probably many medical professionals) over many years, not one of them ever recognized his body odor, kidney stones, or anything else as a symptom of magnesium deficiency. Incredible! This is a good illustration of exactly why so many people all over the world are magnesium deficient. Sadly, no one recognizes it, even when it is right under their nose.

About the Author

Wayne Persky BSME

Wayne Persky was born, grew up, and currently lives in Central Texas. He is a graduate of the University of Texas at Austin, College of Engineering, with postgraduate studies in mechanical engineering, mathematics, and computer science. He has teaching experience in engineering, and business experience in farming and agribusiness.

After the onset of severe digestive system and general health problems in the late 1990s, he went through extensive clinical testing, but the GI specialist failed to take biopsies during a colonoscopy exam, and even failed to test for celiac disease. Afterward, not surprisingly, he was told by his gastroenterologist that there was nothing wrong with him.

Unable to find a medical solution, he was forced to use his research skills to discover innovative ways to resolve his health issues. After extensive study, he identified the likely source of the problem as food sensitivities.

It took a year and a half of avoiding all traces of gluten, plus trial and error experimentation with other foods, and careful record-keeping, to track down all of the food issues. But once he eliminated all of them from his diet, he got his life back. He currently administrates an online microscopic colitis discussion and support forum, while continuing to live on a farm in Central

Why Magnesium Is the Key to Long-Term Health

Texas. In 2015 he founded the Microscopic Colitis Foundation and he continues to serve as president and as a contributing author to the Newsletter.

Contact Details:

Wayne Persky can be contacted at:
Persky Farms
19242 Darrs Creek Rd
Bartlett, TX 76511
USA

Tel: 1(254)718-1125
Tel: 1(254)527-3682

Email: wayne@perskyfarms.com
Email: wayne@microscopiccolitisfoundation.org
Email: wayne@waynepersky.com

For information and support regarding microscopic colitis, visit:

http://www.microscopiccolitisfoundation.org/

To participate in the Discussion and Support Forum go to:

http://www.perskyfarms.com/phpBB2/index.php

My author website can be found at http://www.waynepersky.com/

Why Magnesium Is the Key to Long-Term Health

References

1 Sircus, M. (2009, December 8). Magnesium deficiency symptoms and diagnosis. DrSircus.com. Retrieved from http://drsircus.com/magnesium/magnesium-deficiency-symptoms-diagnosis/

2 Reddy, V., & Sivakumar, B. (1974). Magnesium-dependent vitamin-D-resistant rickets. *The Lancet, 303*(7864), 963–965. Retrieved from http://www.thelancet.com/journals/lancet/article/PIIS0140-6736%2874%2991265-3/abstract

3 Rude, R. K., Adams, J. S., Ryzen, E., Endres, D. B., Niimi, H., Horst, R. L., ... Singer, F. R. (1985). Low serum concentrations of 1,25-dihydroxyvitamin D in human magnesium deficiency. *The Journal of Clinical Endocrinology & Metabolism, 61*(5), 933–940. Retrieved from https://www.ncbi.nlm.nih.gov/pubmed/3840173

4 Takaya, J., Higashino, H., & Kobayashi, Y. (2004). Intracellular magnesium and insulin resistance. *Magnesium Research, 17*(2), 126-136. Retrieved from http://www.ncbi.nlm.nih.gov/pubmed/15319146

5 Sircus, M. (2009, December 8). The Insulin Magnesium Story [Web log message]. Retrieved from http://drsircus.com/medicine/magnesium/the-insulin-magnesium-story-2

6 Hruby, A., Meigs, J. B., O'Donnell, C. J., Jacques, P. F., & McKeown, N. M. (2014). Higher Magnesium Intake Reduces Risk of Impaired Glucose and Insulin Metabolism and Progression From Prediabetes to Diabetes in Middle-Aged

Americans. Diabetes Care, 37(2), 419-427. Retrieved from http://care.diabetesjournals.org/content/37/2/419

7   The chemical secrets of the Mediterranean diet: High levels of magnesium help to reduce risk of strokes, diabetes and heart disease. (Updated 2016, December 8). Retrieved from http://www.dailymail.co.uk/health/article-4011708/The-chemical-secrets-Mediterranean-diet-High-levels-magnesium-help-reduce-risk-strokes-diabetes-heart-disease.html

8   King, D. E., Mainous, A. G. 3rd, Geesey, M. E., & Woolson, R. F. (2005). Dietary magnesium and C-reactive protein levels. *The Journal of The American College of Nutrition*, 24(3), 166-171. Retrieved from https://www.ncbi.nlm.nih.gov/pubmed/15930481

9   Mazur, A., Maier, J. A., Rock, E., Gueux, E., Nowacki, W., & Rayssiguier, Y. (2007). Magnesium and the inflammatory response: potential physiopathological implications. *Archives of Biochemistry and Biophysics*, 458(1), 48–56. Retrieved from https://www.ncbi.nlm.nih.gov/pubmed/16712775

10 Magnesium. (2015, August 06). University of Maryland Medical Center (UMMC). Retrieved from http://www.umm.edu/health/medical/altmed/supplement/magnesium

11 Ma, J., Folsom, A. R., Melnick, S. L., Eckfeldt, J. H., Sharrett, A. R., Nabulsi, A. A., . . . Metcalf, P. A. (1995). Associations of serum and dietary magnesium with cardiovascular disease, hypertension, diabetes, insulin, and carotid arterial wall thickness: the ARIC study. Atherosclerosis Risk in Communities Study. *Journal of Clinical Epidemiology*, 48(7), 927–940. Retrieved from

References

https://www.ncbi.nlm.nih.gov/pubmed/7782801

12 Kiefer, D. (2007, February). Is your bottled water killing you? *Life Extension Magazine.* Retrieved from http://www.lifeextension.com/magazine/2007/2/report_water/Page-01

13 The history of water filters. (n.d.). *Historyofwaterfilters.com.* Retrieved from http://www.historyofwaterfilters.com/

14 Azoulay, A., Garzon, P. & Eisenberg, M. J. (2001). Comparison of the mineral content of tap water and bottled waters. *Journal of General Internal Medicine, 16*(3), 168–175. Retrieved from https://www.ncbi.nlm.nih.gov/pmc/articles/PMC1495189/

15 Liebscher D. H., & Liebscher, D. E. (2004). About the misdiagnosis of magnesium deficiency. *The Journal of the American College of Nutrition, 23*(6), 730S–731S. Retrieved from https://www.ncbi.nlm.nih.gov/pubmed/15637222

16 Touyz, R. M. (2004). Magnesium in clinical medicine. *Frontiers in Bioscience, 1*(9), 1278–1293. Retrieved from https://www.ncbi.nlm.nih.gov/pubmed/14977544

17 Deans, E. (2012, September 11). Is fibromyalgia due to a mineral deficiency? *Psychology Today.* Retrieved from https://www.psychologytoday.com/blog/evolutionary-psychiatry/201209/is-fibromyalgia-due-mineral-deficiency

18 Engen, D. J., McAllister, S. J., Whipple, M. O., Cha, S. S., Dion, L. J., Vincent, A., . . . Wahner-Roedler, D. L. (2015). Effects of transdermal magnesium chloride on quality of life for patients with fibromyalgia: a feasibility study. Journal of Integrative Medicine, 13(5), 306–313. Retrieved from https://www.ncbi.nlm.nih.gov/pubmed/26343101

Why Magnesium Is the Key to Long-Term Health

19 Persky, W. (2013). Vitamin D and Autoimmune Disease. Bartlett, TX: Persky Farms.

20 FDA Drug Safety Communication: (2011, March 2). Low magnesium levels can be associated with long-term use of proton pump inhibitor drugs (PPIs). U.S. Food and Drug Administration [Web log message]. Retrieved from http://www.fda.gov/Drugs/DrugSafety/ucm245011.htm

21 Dean, C. (2015, October 20). Why test for magnesium? [Web log message]. Retrieved from https://drcarolyndean.com/2015/10/why-test-for-magnesium/

22 Magnesium. (n.d.). University of Maryland Medical Center, [Web log message]. Retrieved from http://umm.edu/health/medical/altmed/supplement/magnesium

23 Sircus, M. (2009, December 8). Magnesium thirst magnesium hunger [Web log message]. Retrieved from http://drsircus.com/medicine/magnesium/magnesium-deficiency-symptoms-diagnosis

24 Schachter, M. B. (1996). The importance of magnesium to human nutrition [Web log message]. Retrieved from http://www.mbschachter.com/importance_of_magnesium_to_human.htm

25 Dean, C. (2011, February 20). Magnesium, estrogen and vitamin D. [Web log message]. Retrieved from https://drcarolyndean.

References

26 Zarean, E. & Tarjan, A. (2017). Effect of magnesium supplement on pregnancy outcomes: A randomized control trial. *Advanced Biomedecal Research, 6*, 109. Retrieved from https://www.ncbi.nlm.nih.gov/pmc/articles/PMC5590399/

27 Gilliland, F. D., Berhane K. T., Li, Y. F., Kim, D. H., & Margolis, H. G. (2002). Dietary magnesium, potassium, sodium, and children's lung function. *American Journal of Epidemiology, 155*(2), 125-31. Retrieved from http://www.ncbi.nlm.nih.gov/pubmed/11790675

28 Nuytten, D., Van Hees, J., Meulemans, A., & Carton, H. (1991). Magnesium deficiency as a cause of acute intractable seizures. *Journal of Neurology, 238*(5), 262-264. Retrieved from http://www.ncbi.nlm.nih.gov/pubmed/1919610

29 Yuen, A.W., & Sander, J. W. (2012). Can magnesium supplementation reduce seizures in people with epilepsy? A hypothesis. *Epilepsy Research, 100*(1-2), 152-156. Retrieved from http://www.ncbi.nlm.nih.gov/pubmed/22406257

30 Mauskop, A., & Varughese, J. (2012). Why all migraine patients should be treated with magnesium. *Journal of Neural Transmission (Vienna), 119*(5), 575-579. Retrieved from http://www.ncbi.nlm.nih.gov/pubmed/22426836

31 Galland, L. (1991–1992). Magnesium, stress and neuropsychiatric disorders. *Magnesium and Trace Elements 10*(2-4), 287-301. Retrieved from http://www.ncbi.nlm.nih.gov/pubmed/1844561

32 Eby, G. A., & Eby, K. L. (2006). Rapid recovery from major depression using magnesium treatment. *Medical Hypotheses*, 67(2), 362–370. Retrieved from http://www.ncbi.nlm.nih.gov/pubmed/16542786

33 Ashley (2012, February 10). How Much Magnesium Do I Need? Retrieved from http://www.ancientminerals.com/blog-post/how-much-magnesium/

34 Wang, J., Liu, Y., Zhou, L. J., Wu, Y., Li, F., Shen, K. F., & Liu, X. G. (2013). Magnesium L-threonate prevents and restores memory deficits associated with neuropathic pain by inhibition of TNF-α. *Pain Physician Journal*, 16(5), E563–575. Retrieved from https://www.ncbi.nlm.nih.gov/pubmed/24077207

35 Advantages of magnesium bisglycinate chelate buffered. (n.d.). *Albion Laboratories, Inc.* Retrieved from http://www.albionminerals.com/human-nutrition/magnesium-white-paper

36 Koskela, R. (2011). *Microscopic colitis: Clinical features and gastroduodenal and immunogenic findings.* (Doctoral dissertation, University of Oulu). Retrieved from http://herkules.oulu.fi/isbn9789514294150/isbn9789514294150.pdf

37 DiLauro, S., & Crum-Cianflone, N. F. (2010). Ileitis: When it is not Crohn's disease. *Current Gastroenterology Reports*, 12(4), 249–258. Retrieved from https://www.ncbi.nlm.nih.gov/pmc/articles/PMC2914216/

38 Cojocaru, I. M., Cojocaru, M., Tănăsescu, R., Iacob, S. A., & Iliescu, I. (2009). Changes of magnesium serum levels in

References

patients with acute ischemic stroke and acute infections. *Romanian Journal of Internal Medicine*, 47(2), 169–671. Retrieved from https://www.ncbi.nlm.nih.gov/pubmed/20067167

39 Kent, L. T. (2015, November 11). Hashimoto's and magnesium deficiency. *Livestrong.com*. Retrieved from http://www.livestrong.com/article/547017-hashimotos-and-magnesium-deficiency/

40 Keefer, A. (2017, October 3). What beverages are high in magnesium and phosphorus? Retrieved from https://www.livestrong.com/article/529466-what-beverages-are-high-in-magnesium-and-phosphorus/

41 Nishio, A., Ishiguro, S., & Miyao, N. (1987). Specific change of histamine metabolism in acute magnesium-deficient young rats. *Drug Nutrient Interactions*, 5(2), 89-96. Retrieved from https://www.ncbi.nlm.nih.gov/pubmed/3111814

42 Dolhun, R. (2014, December 08). Gut check on Parkinson's: New findings on bacteria levels. Retrieved from https://www.michaeljfox.org/foundation/news-detail.php?gut-check-on-parkinson-new-findings-on-bacteria-levels

43 Kwon, K. Y., Jo, K. D., Lee, M. K., Oh, M, Kim, E. N., Park, J.,. . . . Jang, W. (2016). Low serum vitamin D levels may contribute to gastric dysmotility in de novo Parkinson's disease. *Neurodegenerative Diseases*, 16(3-4),199-205. Retrieved from https://www.ncbi.nlm.nih.gov/pubmed/26735311

44 Golts, N., Snyder, H., Frasier, M., Theisler, C., Choi, P., & Wolozin, B. (2002). Magnesium inhibits spontaneous and iron-induced aggregation of alpha-synuclein. *Journal of Biolog-*

ical Chemistry, 277(18), 16116–16123. Retrieved from http://www.jbc.org/content/277/18/16116.long

45 Guo, J. L., Covell, D. J., Daniels, J. P., Iba, M., Stieber, A., Zhang, B., & Lee, V. M. (2013). Distinct α-synuclein strains differentially promote tau inclusions in neurons. Cell Journal, 154(1),103–117. Retrieved from https://www.ncbi.nlm.nih.gov/pmc/articles/PMC3820001/

46 Jones, R. (2013, May 27). Magnesium supplement to treat alzheimer's disease. Knowing Neurons. [Web log message]. Retrieved from https://knowingneurons.com/2013/05/27/magnesium-supplement-to-treat-alzheimers-disease/

47 Fischer, K. (2017, September 21). Why it matters whether you're getting enough magnesium. [Web log message]. Retrieved from http://www.sheknows.com/health-and-wellness/articles/1009485/more-magnesium-for-hormonal-balance

48 Dibaba, D., Xun, P., Yokota, K., White, E., & He, K. (2015). Magnesium intake and incidence of pancreatic cancer: The VITamins and Lifestyle study. *British Journal of Cancer, 113*(11), 1612–1621. Retrieved from http://www.ncbi.nlm.nih.gov/pubmed/26554653

49 Magnesium Fact Sheet for Health Professionals. (2016, February 11). National Institutes of Health Office of Dietary Supplements [Web log message]. Retrieved from https://ods.od.nih.gov/factsheets/Magnesium-HealthProfessional/

References

50 Gardner, T. B. (n.d.). Pancreatic neuroendocrine tumors [Web log message]. The National Pancreas Foundation. Retrieved from https://www.pancreasfoundation.org/patient-information/pancreatic-cancer/pancreatic-neuroendocrine-tumors/

51 McDougall, J. (2011, November). Why did Steve Jobs die? The McDougall Newsletter [Web log message]. Retrieved from https://www.drmcdougall.com/misc/2011nl/nov/jobs.htm

52 Liu, H., Huang, D., McArthur, D. L., Boros, L. G., Nissen, N., & Heaney, A. P. (2010). Fructose induces transketolase flux to promote pancreatic cancer growth. *Cancer Research, 79*(15), 6,368–6,376. Retrieved from http://cancerres.aacrjournals.org/content/70/15/6368.long

53 Ancira, K. (updated 2018, April 06). What is the difference between sucrose, glucose & fructose? Healthy Eating [Web log message]. Retrieved from http://healthyeating.sfgate.com/difference-between-sucrose-glucose-fructose-8704.html

54 Mertz, R. (2014, January 6). Did you know that Steve Jobs became vegan because he believed the diet would... [Web log message]. Retrieved from http://www.tydknow.com/did-you-know-that-steve-jobs-became-vegan-because-he-believed-the-diet-would/

www.ingramcontent.com/pod-product-compliance
Lightning Source LLC
Chambersburg PA
CBHW071122030426
42336CB00013BA/2167